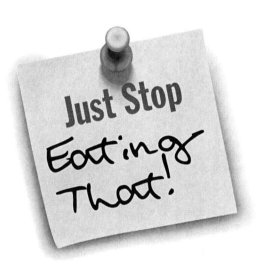

The Rapid Advance Process
to Stop Overeating

Ellie Izzo, PhD and
Vicki Carpel Miller, BSN, MS, LMFT

Just Stop Eating That!

Published by:
HCI Press
7701 E. Indian School Rd. Ste. F
Scottsdale, AZ 85251 USA
www.hcipress.com

A Note to the Reader: The information, ideas and suggestions in this book are not intended as a substitute for professional advice. Before following any suggestions contained in this book you should consult your personal physician or mental health professional. Neither the authors nor the publisher shall be liable or responsible for any loss or damage allegedly arising as a consequence of your use or application of any information or suggestions in this book.

Library of Congress Control Number: 2011938831

ISBN-10: 1-936268-23-X
ISBN-13: 978-1-936268-23-8

High Conflict Institute Press
Scottsdale, Arizona

PRESS

Book Design by www.KarrieRoss.com
Images from istockphoto.com

ALSO BY ELLIE IZZO AND VICKI CARPEL MILLER

Second-Hand Shock: Surviving & Overcoming Vicarious Trauma
Just Stop Doing That
Just Stop Picking Losers

ALSO BY ELLIE IZZO

The Bridge To I Am

CONTENTS

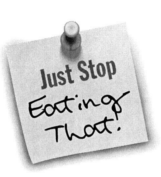

What's Eating You?

Munching Mary

It had been one very long night, with two bags of kettle cooked potato chips, a pint of mocha almond ice cream, and two boxes of double-stuffed Oreo cookies, all washed down with a liter of Cherry Coke. And, still, Mary found herself pawing through the pantry in search of more sugary treats.

Throughout the day Mary would eat healthy meals, but when the sun set, her self-control melted. Her nightly binges left her tipping the scales at 275 pounds, overwhelming her petite frame and height. After each binge, an exhausted and devastated Mary would drop onto her bed, bury her head in her pillow and cry. After a few hours of restless sleep, she would awaken, ashamed, and brace herself for another day of eating her heart out.

Obesity is a disease that takes its toll on a person physically, emotionally, mentally and spiritually. It is devastatingly isolating and lonely. Health experts deem it one of the most significant health problems for children and adults in the world. It doesn't take much research to find that obesity is at an all-time high.

In the United States alone, approximately fifty-eight million people are overweight, forty million are obese, and three million are morbidly obese (reference?). The problem contributes to approximately 80% of Type II Diabetes, 70% of cardiovascular disease, 42% of breast and colon cancer cases, and 26% of high blood pressure cases. Statistics on childhood obesity indicate that over twenty-two million of the world's children under five years of age carry an unhealthy amount of extra weight.

If you've ever spoken with a person struggling with a weight problem, you'd find that most of them have been on numerous diets, have even lost hundreds of pounds, and still battle an eating habit that directly threatens their precious lives. Most of all, they are broken-hearted and sad about themselves. The good news is that research is beginning to discover that many people's brains are actually 'hard-wired' in childhood to binge eat. How and when does that happen? Can you even begin to address that type of challenge? We say, "YES!" with the help of the five simple steps of the Rapid Advance Process.

Change, especially changing bad habits, is hard — and rightly so, as any neuroscientist will tell you. Advances in neuroimaging have enabled researchers to peer inside the brains of people with addictive behaviors. They can see, in real-time, what gets people hooked. They observe how the brain's reward system—based largely on the neurotransmitter dopamine—thirsts for more, while inhibitory control centers experience a system failure. What this means in plain English is that you become addicted to the chemicals your brain emits while you are binge eating, causing your will power (your control center) to fail.

The pattern is similar across all kinds of behaviors—from cocaine and tobacco addiction to overeating. That's why changing your mind may be the first step toward breaking a habit. The brains "machinery" actually changes.

That's why changing your mind may be the first step toward breaking a habit.

Under normal circumstances, dopamine plays a major role in motivation and reward, surging before and during a pleasurable activity—say, eating or sex—to make people want to repeat a behavior that's crucial to the survival of the species. In order for humans to survive, we have to be nourished and we have to reproduce. People who struggle with binge eating are struggling with a motivation and reward system spun out of control.

Dopamine travels in pathways between the brains' limbic system and hippocampus. The limbic system is the center of our emotional reactions. The hippocampus is the relay station for storing and retrieving memories. This combination etches rewarding behaviors into the brain with strong, even seductive, memories.

The problem arises when the memory and the craving to recapture it take over a person's life. The need to experience the pleasure of dopamine and the repetition of doing it creates a pathway that is as wide as a freeway with no exits in sight.

These high-jacked pleasure reward pathways take a formidable stronghold on our brains and our whole existence when they're so closely connected physiologically and anatomically with our memories and our emotions. As the dopamine surge gains speed, the brakes fail. Normal function in the brain's frontal lobes, which are responsible for self-control and executive functioning, (will power) tends to decrease in people who become addicted to the dopamine rush. Can you believe it?! It's not actually the food that pleases you, but the dopamine rush that eating triggers in your brain.

To overcome binge eating, you must find a way to shift your neurological firing away from the hijacked pleasure reward pathways that push you to want to overeat. You can then redirect the firing to the pathways that lead to the frontal lobes of your brain, which will allow you to inhibit (stop) the addictive behavior. How can you do this when the reward is so pleasurable? That's the million dollar question!

Can you imagine what it would be like or what you would give for the opportunity to reframe your relationship with food so that it no longer takes over your willpower, threatens your life, your self-esteem and peace of mind? The ability to build neural pathways to the higher mind and to responsible eating can be achieved through the five simple steps of the *Rapid Advance Process.*

The Five Steps of the Rapid Advance Process

RELINQUISHMENT of JUDGMENT	THOUGHT OF PEACE
1. **Reveal Your History**	*It happened.* It was
2. **Recognize Your Impasse**	*It is still happening.* It is.
3. **Release Your Past**	*I can forgive.* I can.
4. **Respond to Your Fear**	*I stop and look within.* I know.
5.**Reconnect to Your Spirit**	*I find myself.* I am.

These five simple steps to emotional growth and physical health empower you to move out of hard-wired, primitive brain, fear-based thinking and forge new, strong neural pathways to the higher mind or spiritual perspective. Living life from the higher mind empowers you to control your impulses around food.

Remarkably, this 'mindfulness' is achieved by uncovering and forgiving old childhood heartbreaks—the historical hurts that lurk in the unconscious mind and secretly thwart you from having a balanced relationship with food. Through working the five simple steps of the *Rapid Advance Process*, you will quickly arrive at an "Aha!" moment as you achieve forgiveness and release the heavy, buried burdens of times gone by. You will find relief from your underlying fear of being inadequate and shift into using food to nourish your body, rather than binge with it to fill a perceived void.

Overeating is a bad habit among many other difficult-to-break patterns. If you read our first book in this series, **Just Stop Doing That!**, you will remember that some bad habits are easier than others to stop, but all of them have their roots in your deepest fears. Funny, but when you think about the bad habit of overeating, fear is the last thing that comes to your mind because eating tends to bring you some false sense of comfort or relief. Eating whatever you want whenever you want may make you feel better for awhile, but the devastating shame spiral soon follows. Then you eat some more. And some more. Overeating is a dangerous cycle. It is dangerous not only because of the health risks involved but also because while you are binging, you are actively disconnecting from the power of your spirit. You are suffocating your true self with layers of unwanted fat and draining yourself from your motivation to live a joyful life.

Completing the five simple steps of the Rapid Advance Process will help you:

- **Identify your true hunger**
- **Unravel how your history with food has turned you into an eating machine**
- **Reframe your relationship with food**
- **Triumph over your deepest fears**
- **Rediscover your confidence and independence**
- **Choose empowerment and joy for fulfillment**

CHAPTER ONE

What in Heaven's Name Happened to You?

Step One: Reveal Your History

Franny the Freshman

They told Franny it was the freshman fifteen—those extra fifteen pounds many incoming freshmen were reputed to gain as they launched into campus living. But that was over thirty pounds ago and she had yet to begin her second semester. Franny, superficially, appeared to have made a smooth transition into dorm life. She had friends and did extremely well in her class-es. Yet she still felt a loneliness from time to time that rattled her soul. That's when she would turn to food for comfort. She would order a large pizza and eat the whole thing, she'd drink a liter of beer to ease her pain and she swallowed M&Ms by the pound-size bag. She was eating her heart out.

By the beginning of her sophomore year, Franny had gained over 40 pounds. Two years later, at her college graduation, she had put on over 130 pounds. When her health became endangered from diabetes, she found us and started the Rapid Advance Process. In that process she began to reveal her history.

She saw herself as a happy little girl until her parents divorced when she was six years old. Her father walked out. Years would go by between visits. Her mother worked hard to make up for the loss and on a conscious level, Franny had no awareness of her deeply hidden, little-girl fear that if her mother walked out as well, she would be abandoned and could die. That kind of fear was way over-the-top for a six-year-old. As a result, Franny swallowed her fear with food. Her years in soccer helped her burn the extra calories, but she stopped playing sports when she started college.

Franny's old fear and loneliness got triggered when she separated from her Mom to attend college. It was her fear of abandonment that drove her need to distract herself by binging. Obesity became her protective cushion between herself and her lonesome fear that had its roots in an earlier time.

Losing the Baby Fat

Your first response to the question, "What in heaven's name happened to you?" may be, "Nothing." We wouldn't be surprised if your answer was exactly that. That's why you chow down rather than look within and face your demons. Your distraction of overeating keeps you estranged from your history or as we call it, your personal truth. We're not saying that your history is all bad, but the good stuff isn't of much interest right now. We're only interested in identifying when you first started feeling afraid.

> *Your distraction of overeating keeps*
> *you estranged from your history ...*
> *your personal truth.*

You didn't come into this world feeling afraid. You were born a little ball of love, precious and innocent until life started happening to you. Your ego, or the personality you show the world, began developing as a defense against feeling afraid. This happens to everyone to some degree. All children feel afraid about something at some point. It doesn't have to be a big, catastrophic event. Different things impact different children in different ways. For example, some little kids love to ride roller coasters while other kids are terrified.

Whether your fears from childhood are rooted in memories of:

- being sent to bed without dinner
- a dark closet, being accosted by a scary child
- being caught in the rain
- coming home from school and having no one in the house
- being forced to eat all your dinner
- being disciplined
- hearing strange noises
- having nightmares
- losing a friend
- losing a love
- going through a divorce
- being forced to eat food you didn't like
- having an accident
- feeling publicly embarrassed in school or in front of the family
- becoming ill and missing out on important activities
- shyness in school
- moving a lot

These memories are stored. When these historical feeling states are triggered by something in the present, you are at risk to turn to your overeating as a way to cope. We believe there is an alternative.

You may think that your personal childhood history holds no triggers or truly upsetting events, but in reality, your childhood holds the key to how your brain became hard-wired for overeating. Many of us have forgotten much of the past or perhaps have developed a selective recall about it. We are not suggesting that you get bogged down in your past, but reviewing it has merit. This review provides an opportunity to use your history as a catalyst to make positive brain-changes in the here and now and **Just Stop Eating That!**

The ability to respond to fear is necessary to adequately cope with life's many stressors.

We are interested in how your judgment or perception of some of your historical events may have caused a break, or as we call it, an Impasse, to your higher thinking or spiritual perspective. Because you were afraid, you distracted yourself with something pleasurable to take your mind away from the fear. This pleasurable distraction released dopamine in your brain and created an embedded pathway that becomes overused. This fear, or Impasse, hard-wired your brain to automatically override your own proficient will-power and, instead, seeks the pathway of pleasure.

This scenario keeps you stuck and unable to reach your higher thinking–the ability that empowers you to control your impulses and directly respond to feeling afraid. The ability to respond to fear is necessary to adequately cope with life's many stressors. When the pathway to your higher mind is blocked, or develops an Impasse, you "hit the wall" and have no choice other than to retreat back into an old nagging fear that keeps you trapped in the distracting, impulsive part of your thinking. So after you hit the wall, you hit the fridge and impulsively turn to food to distract and falsely soothe yourself.

Hungry Hannah

Hannah was an over-eater. She was hungry all the time. She tried to curb her appetite, but when she started to eat, she simply could not stop. She boasted that she never met a meal she didn't like. She also boasted that she had lost thousands of pounds over the course of her adult life by going on trendy diets, but always managed to gain the weight back and then some. At thirty-two years old and 283 pounds, Hannah was broken-hearted and wanting a change.

Hannah was an only child. When Hannah was young, she witnessed a lot of fighting between her parents. Her father would end up storming out of the house and be gone for many hours, and sometimes for days. Her mother would retreat into her bedroom and close the door. After what seemed to Hannah to be hours of sobbing, all would go quiet and her mom would remain sequestered in her bedroom for many hours. She felt alone and afraid.

Needless to say, she spent a lot of time by herself. She remembers knocking on her mother's bedroom door very quietly and receiving no response. That would frighten her, but she was even more afraid of knocking harder and upsetting her mother even more. So she would go into the kitchen and indulge in way too much food in between her periods of quiet knocking on her mother's door.

By the time Hannah entered first grade, she was thirty pounds overweight. Her parents told her, "Stop eating all that junk food, Hannah. You're really getting chubby." Hannah could tell that her parents were embarrassed about her appearance, but comforting herself during their conflicts by overeating had a strong-hold on Hannah as a self-soothing behavior or distraction. As an adult, Hannah found it hard to ever be alone, and continued to swallow her fear in food.

Just like Hannah, when you were a child and started to feel afraid, you developed your Impasses—those road-blocks to the neural pathways that take you to your spiritual perspective or higher thinking. Fear created Impasses for you and arrested your ability to connect to the precious higher state of your innocence. Soothing or distracting behaviors, such as overeating, led you into a compulsive behavior that was and continues to be hurt-ful to you. This repetitive behavior was, at the time, actually good in that it helped you survive and relieved your feelings of fear. How ironic is it that survival behaviors of childhood can become life threatening as we grow!

A child typically looks to a parent to help with their fears, but sometimes it is the parent who is causing the fear. Maybe your parents didn't realize that you were scared. They may have reacted to your distracting behaviors with criticism or neglect, as we saw with Hannah. It is of no use to you to blame your parents. It is time for you to take control of your own life. And, don't forget, just like everyone else, your parents were operating with their own assorted distractions to remain unconscious of their childhood fears which had nothing whatsoever to do with you.

> *How ironic is it that survival behaviors*
> *of childhood can become life*
> *threatening as we grow!*

Many parents become focused on their child's distracting behavior, thinking the behavior itself is the problem, when, in fact, it is the child's *solution* to feeling afraid. It is the *only* way the child can cope with the fear or the Impasse. The child simply does not yet have the brain or intellectual development to handle it differently. As a child, when you are young and afraid, it is easy to stay in that addictive loop of dopamine. After all, a child's higher brain is not developed or fully functional until the early to mid twenties, typically around age 25. By the time your higher brain is in place, the negative loop already has its stronghold on you.

It's Not All in Your Mind—It's All in Your Brain

We don't want to go too scientific on you, but it is very important that you have an understanding of the human brain's involvement in overeating. People who have incorporated bad habits into their lives operate in a fear-driven, mid-brain circuitry. The "overeating" brain circuit burrows deeply and repetitively into the gray matter until it starts to resemble the configuration of a freeway, deeply grooved and six lanes wide. Never-ending with no exits. With each repetition of the binge eating, the grooves in the road get deeper and more entrenched and the possibilities of getting off the freeway are considerably less.

As you grow, your brain continues to develop within the delicate balance between your genetics and your environment, continuously impacted by your experiences.

"Binge eating neurons" race around the loop, making pit stops at the addiction receptors to refuel with more food. They never get off the road. Our goal is to get your brain to work more effectively by forging strong pathways to your higher mind where fear can be faced and overcome with healthy thinking first, and then, healthy eating.

When was the last time you had a good look at your brain? We want you to have an elementary and enlightening observation of your brain so you might better understand some of the scientific dynamics of how this works. Your brain developed rapidly within the early years of life. Some experts believe that the stage was set for your personality by the time you were five years old. As you grow, your brain continues to develop within the delicate balance between your genetics and your environment, continuously impacted by your experiences.

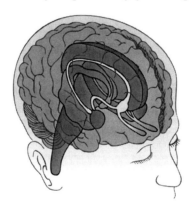

As babies, we all start out with a primitive brain: we eat, sleep and poop. These are considered to be automatic, instinctual brain functions. The almond-shaped structure in the mid/lower brain is called the amygdale and is the center of your basic instincts of flight, fight, or freeze. This is the part of our brain that we share with all animals.

The amygdale is responsible for basic survival and gets your body ready to immediately react when you feel afraid. The magnet-shaped hippocampus, or as we good-naturedly call it, "the hippo", is the relay station of our brain. When you have an experience, good or bad, a memory is created and stored in your brain. Throughout your life, relationships and events may trigger those stored memories. The hippo retrieves and replays those memories for you. You then relive these memories. This can be great, or at times, it can be very daunting. Never underestimate the control and power of the hippo!

Look at the picture again. The hippo is connected to the amygdale. When a painful memory is retrieved and replayed by the hippo, the basic instinctual feelings of fear around that memory get triggered as well. The present day event doesn't have to be an exact match to the memory; it could be as basic as a similar smell, a taste, a sound, a word or an action.

When you are very young and unaware, all the scary stuff of life is happening to you and that stuff gets stored in your brain. The hippocampus can magnetize these memories to the forefront and then the amygdale trigger the instinctual flight, fight or freeze reaction. The power of the hippo triggers you to choose the "flight" reaction of overeating as your distraction from feeling some old, nagging fear.

The outer area of the brain is the cortex and develops as we grow into adulthood. The cerebral cortex or the intellect/higher mind begins to grow as we grow. This growth includes the development of neural pathways which resemble the configuration of an organic switch-board. Certain areas of the brain become stimulated as we experience the environment. The more certain areas are stimulated, the stronger the connecting neural pathway grows and the deeper it settles into the gray matter.

Hopefully, with healthy development, we build a neuro-infrastructure that helps us to use our higher brain, to navigate away from basic instincts of fight, flight or freeze so that we might *respond* in appropriate situations rather than *react*. We grow into adulthood developing the ability to switch into calmer, higher thinking as a more evolved way to handle stress. Some of us have developed this ability better than others. Have you ever heard the phrase, "His brain is just not 'wired' that way?" What do you think that means? There is a lack of 'wiring' in the immature neuron.

When the neural pathways to your higher mind or spiritual perspective are immature, underused or under-developed, you may find yourself at what we call the Impasse—that place where you cannot easily access your higher, calmer mind. Neurologically, you hit the wall, and then the fridge, and become trapped in lower brain thinking. This thinking is based more on instincts of fight, flight or freeze and is driven by an unrecognized fear. You feel separated and alone. The more you eat, the more alone you feel.

This repetition is really scary and reinforces the flawed, underlying motivation to seek out food and swallow the upset rather than relying on your own internal resources. If you take one cup of your brain development; add to it 2 tablespoons of how food was approached in your childhood; add a quarter cup of your sub-conscious memory; add a pinch of your parents' traits or characteristics, and you will have a foolproof recipe for a very fattening dish.

The emotional blueprint from your childhood has set the stage for your habit of overeating as an adult. We wonder if you can imagine yourself turning to courage, faith, and hope instead of food? We believe that the emptiness or the perceived void you try to fill with food is simply the loneliness you experience as a result of being disconnected from your spirit.

The emotional blueprint from your childhood has set the stage for your habit of overeating as an adult.

Reconnecting to your spiritual perspective is a far more effective way to rise above your fears in life. If you find yourself stuck in repetitive eating habits, consider how it is that you have forgotten about the power of your higher mind or have become disconnected from your spirit. It is only by accessing the higher mind that you truly overcome your fears, stop your overeating and experience satisfaction and peace in your daily life.

We don't want anything from you except your willingness to move through the five simple steps of the Rapid Advance Process, with the goal of stopping your overeating. Not only will you have the opportunity to stop, but you will start receiving something far more nourishing and satisfying instead.

We suspect that the thought of stopping your overeating is scary in and of itself. If you are tired of being a slave to food, if you are weary with people who care about you complaining and begging you to stop, we want to help you. We believe that this little book with our five simple steps has the ability to do so. Imagine yourself choosing not to eat as you stand in front of the opened refrigerator? Think about driving right past the fast food restaurant. Picture yourself recognizing your desire to binge in advance of acting it out and instead, taking the desire to do so in a different direction. You would be in control of your habit! It would no longer be in control of you!

Once you have recognized what you are afraid of, you can rid yourself of your binging and stop eating your heart out!

How would you feel if you knew that your overeating isn't really your problem? That, instead, it is a distraction from something else far easier to overcome than the overeating itself? Our goal is to help you discover your personal Impasse, or break, from your essence or spirit; that point in your early experience where you began to feel afraid. Once you have recognized what you are afraid of, you can rid yourself of your binging and stop eating your heart out! Now, let's get to work.

Get a journal or pad of paper and get ready to start writing your story. Start as early as you can remember and write statements about your childhood, your family, your school, your friends and anything significant that happened to you. Write your history as if it were a narrative or story. Take your time. Pay attention and don't leave stuff out. Below are some action items to help you complete your story.

Take Action: Growing Up You

Describe your early memories of your mother's personality with five adjectives, e.g. caring, critical, judgment, loving, etc.:

1. _____
2. _____
3. _____
4. _____
5. _____

Describe your early memories of your father's personality with five adjectives:

1. _____
2. _____
3. _____
4. _____
5. _____

Did your family suffer a life-altering event such as a death or divorce? How was this addressed?

_____

_____

_____

If you lived in a blended family system, please describe the dynamics associated with this experience.

_____

_____

_____

Action Items

Describe your parents' marriage with five adjectives.

1. _____

2. _____

3. _____

4. _____

5. _____

How did your parents/stepparents resolve their conflicts? What did you see? What did you hear or not hear?

_____

_____

_____

How did you feel when your parents/step-parents were having conflicts?

_____

_____

_____

How did you feel when conflicts went unaddressed?

_____

_____

_____

How did your parents/step-parents handle issues around money?

_____

_____

_____

How did your parents/step-parents handle issues around religion?

_____

_____

_____

How did your family have fun together?

_____

_____

_____

How was affection displayed in your family?

_____

_____

_____

How were issues around sex approached in your family?

_____

_____

_____

How was illness addressed in your family?

_____

_____

_____

Was there any addiction or substance abuse in your family? How did it you affect you?

_____

_____

_____

What was the role of extended family? Were you close to Aunts, Uncles, and cousins?

_____

_____

_____

How were you disciplined?

_____

_____

_____

How were your relationships with your siblings? What was your birth order?

_____

_____

_____

How did your parents/step-parents handle issues around food?

_____

_____

_____

When did you first start to over eat? What was happening at the time?

_____

_____

_____

What was the meaning of food in your household?

_____

_____

_____

What were the myths and stories you would hear around eating and food?

_____

_____

_____

Were events around food or eating ever used as discipline? Explain.

_____

_____

_____

Were you ever rewarded with food? Explain.

_____

_____

_____

Were your parents obese or binge eaters?

_____

_____

_____

Did your parents hoard food? Explain.

_____

_____

_____

Do you have any awareness of your parents' history around food? Explain.

_____

_____

_____

Did your parents have awareness and education about nutrition? If so, what did they teach you about it?

_____

_____

_____

Were you a fast food baby? Explain why and how.

_____

_____

_____

Was food a substitute for something else? If so, what?

_____

_____

_____

This **Action Plan** of **Revealing Your History** has awakened your personal truth about the story of your life. You may be beginning to notice some themes and patterns that make you curious to know more. Becoming aware and intimate with your past helps bring you back to your power to reframe it in a healing and helpful way so that it does not play out 'sideways' in your present day relationship with food.

CHAPTER TWO

Hitting the Fridge

Step Two: Recognize Your Impasse

Dining Don

Don was lost in his world of obesity. He had no secure job, no secure relationship and no strategy for taking care of himself. He had been married three times to three abusive women. The first wife was a drug addict; the second wife was invisible because she was so intimidated by his size; and his third wife was completely aloof and disconnected from him. He found himself alone much of the time and food was his main companion.

He was a bright enough person, but his binge eating had taken hold of his life and nothing he tried seemed to

*work. Even the gastric bypass surgery he endured ten
years ago was not enough to stop his compulsion to eat.
He had gained and lost hundreds of pounds in the course
of his forty-four years.*

*Historically, Don was always chubby. He was raised
by a dominating mother and a very passive, compliant
father. His mother demanded that he eat and was down-
right overbearing in her approach to food. Mealtime was
the only source of family connection and, unfortunately,
it was much more about the food and not really about
the connection. If he didn't eat his mother's meals, she
perceived that he was rejecting her love and she would
punish him for that by dropping the curtain of silence.
He would sometimes sit at the table for hours with his
spinach sitting in front of him. Other times he would
even fall asleep at the table.*

*Don felt unloved during these periods of power-strug-
gling around food and he learned early on that cleaning
his plate was the only way to be safe and feel loved.*

When Don revealed his history, it was obvious that
food presented an emotional impasse for him in that he
could identify it as a substitute for healthy love. His fear
was that if he didn't overeat, he would be abandoned by
his mother and die. Ironically, he lived out this fear over
and over again, by abandoning himself through his
distraction of compulsive overeating.

As a child, he was afraid to refuse food lest he be
abandoned and so he judged himself as unlovable to his

mother just as he was—a cute little kid who didn't really have that big of an appetite. His brothers and sister were taller and thinner and could metabolize food much more quickly than he. Don distracted himself from his Impasse of fear of abandonment by overeating. The vicious cycle was that the more he overate and the bigger he got, he generated more and more self-loathing. Don wanted to find another way to approach this challenge in his life. Don wanted to face the challenge of changing his brain and how it operated in regards to food.

The Origins of Impasse

Revealing your history and then recognizing your impasse is paramount to changing your overeating. The habit of binge eating is actually not the problem; it is a person's solution or distraction from the real problem. We call the real problem your Impasse.

Your Impasse can sometimes be very difficult to put into words. It is difficult because it is rooted so early in your life, it may present itself as a weird feeling or a body memory. It may have originally set in at a time when you did not possess the verbal development to speak about it. But we promise you, it is in there and you need to identify and make friends with it. Your habit of overeating is nothing more than a distraction or avoidance of your fear. You can't fix if you can't find it.

So let's work on identifying your Impasse and let's start by giving it some definition. Your Impasse is an emotional and physical fear reaction that has its roots in your history. Your Impasse is three-dimensional. It includes your memory of a painful event. It includes your feelings at the time of the event. It also includes how you judged yourself and others in the context of the event.

Let's apply this to Don. His memory of the painful event was that he was forced to clean his plate or else his mom would be angry at him. His feelings at the time of the event were fear and sadness. He was afraid that he would be abandoned and he was sad that his mother didn't appear to love him. His judgment of himself was that he must be unlovable or unacceptable unless he ate it all up. As long as he kept eating, it would all be okay. This made Don feel better and therefore provided him pleasure. Don's brain became hardwired in this continuous loop and his challenge was to redesign his neural pathways so that his eating behaviors could be regulated from his higher thinking instead of being regulated from his more primitive limbic system.

Mac 'n Cheese Mona

Mona was the second-born in a family with an older brother who was greatly revered by her parents. Her older brother could do no wrong in their eyes and he played that role to an academy award-winning performance. He would berate Mona on the sly, but behave beautifully with her when the parents were within earshot. Mona used to feel hopeless as a child. She alternated between feeling either invisible to her parents or abused by her brother. It all added up to some very poor self esteem and feelings of extreme loneliness.

Mona's older brother got all the attention and she was basically ignored. She tried to be perfect as an attempt to fix it. If she was perfect, maybe then she would be loved. She got straight A's, had popular friends, and always looked perfectly together, but it was still never enough to get the acceptance of her parents.

The turning point for her physically was when she tried out for volleyball and didn't make it. She attributed the loss to being underweight, even though she was average in size. With that event, Mona's attention became hyper-focused to food and the faulty thinking that if she were bigger, then she would be noticed. And she got bigger and bigger and bigger. She also got noticed, but in a negative way. "You're fat!" her mother would cry. "What is happening to you?" her father would ask. Mona finally started getting noticed alright by her parents, but with some very negative attention.

The piece de resistance was when Mona redecorated her room by covering one of the walls with Mac and Cheese boxes. Her parents were appalled and demanded that she keep the door to her room closed at all times.

Things continued to spin out of control when Mona began to let boys cross her boundaries sexually in order to feel some love and affection. But too much food and too much sex only made her feel worse. Mona was on a neurological crash course and she needed to change her mind about herself.

Let's practice recognizing the Impasse by looking at Mona's story. Her memory of a painful event was that she was ignored by her parents while her brother was put on a pedestal. Her feelings at the time of this event were fear and sadness: fear that she would be alone and sadness that she was invisible to the two most important people in her life—her parents.

Her judgment of herself in the context of this event was that she must be unlovable and inadequate because she was not worthy of being seen. As long as she kept eating, she would be noticed. This made Mona feel better and therefore provided her pleasure. Mona's brain became hardwired in this continuous loop and her challenge was to redesign her neural pathways so that her eating behaviors could be regulated from her higher thinking instead of being regulated from her more primitive limbic system.

Mouthful Mark

Mark was a change-of-life baby. He was the apple strudel of his mother's eye. She loved his toddler pudginess and spent lots of time with him doing fun things. His father would take him to the office and show him off to staff and work while Mark played on the floor next to the big desk. Mark loved his daddy and life was great, until his father died unexpectedly from a massive stroke. Mark never got to say goodbye.

Everything changed dramatically after Mark's dad died. There was no life insurance and his Mom had to return to work as a nurse. Her father-in-law agreed to be supportive by financing Mark's education at a high-end boarding school. So, at the innocent age of

10 years old, Mark found himself in the scary halls of his new school, hundreds of miles from home, alone and disliked by his classmates.

In his first few weeks, Mark was bullied and perpetrated upon by a group of older boys. They forced him to wear a blindfold and threw him in a pool full of filthy water. He almost drowned. To make matters worse, the teachers and administrators did nothing to intervene or protect him. He was afraid to tell his mother and grandfather because he did not want to be a disappointment to them.

The only place that was safe haven for Mark was the dining hall. There was a strict code of behavior there and Mark could enjoy long periods of solace and sanctuary as long as he was eating. Needless to say, he was eating a lot and managed to gain sixty-five pounds in one year.

Mark returned home the following year and went back to public school. His attachment to the comfort of food persisted even though his environment greatly improved. He felt like he was a disappointment to his family because he couldn't fit in at boarding school. He felt burdened by the loss of his father and a perceived pressure to take care of his mother so that she wouldn't die like Dad. He just ate and ate and ate.

Mark was using food to comfort any level of anxiety or distress he felt, particularly when he thought about being a disappointment to his family. His memory of a painful event was that he lost his childhood with the death of his father. His feelings at the time of the event were fear and sadness. He was afraid of being a disappointment to his mother and sad at the loss of his precious Dad and the loss of his innocence.

His judgment of himself in the context of this event was that he must be unlovable and unacceptable because he was a disappointment. This became his Impasse and binge eating was Mark's distraction from his heavy feeling of inadequacy.

It Really Has A Hold On You!

Look at the underlying and silent themes from **Revealing Your History** to help you recognize your Impasse. Many times these themes appear subtle and unimportant from a grown-up point-of-view. For example, in some families, boys are treated differently than girls. In other families, some religious practices crowd out healthy and direct communication. Money issues, changing values, and family secrets can all contribute to creating Impasses.

In recognizing your Impasse, don't

always look for the obvious.

In other situations, how others saw the family might have been more important than what was truly happening within it. In recognizing your Impasse, don't always look for the obvious. Many times it is the unspoken themes or codes of silence that can drive the Impasse forward, sometimes for generations.

Once you recognize your Impasse, you might notice that you feel anxious. We think this is separation anxiety. Separation anxiety is commonly thought of as the upset a child feels when he or she must detach from a parent. Consider this thought—what if separation anxiety is actually the chronic underlying distress you feel as a result of being separated from the most loving and nurturing spiritual part of YOURSELF? If this is true, we remain separated by fear in adulthood and stuff our faces as a way to avoid feeling this unpleasant anxiety. Imagine what might happen if you were to recognize and then meet this anxiety head on. Then, maybe your eating behaviors would look very different.

What You Really Think of You

When a child perceives that he/she did not get the unconditional acceptance needed from either parent, a part of them never really quite matures and individuates. They look grown up and in a lot of ways they act grown up, but somewhere in their subconscious is a frightened little child who craves this love. This little child can pop up at any time, just like a jack-in-the box, trying to complete this perceived missing part of their development and calm themselves down from anxiety. Filling the void and feeling better becomes mistakenly addressed by impulsively and compulsively overeating, but that behavior only makes matters worse. You probably already know how awful you feel about yourself after a binge.

Re-creating the Impasse has an addictive quality to it...

Re-creating the Impasse has an addictive quality to it; the familiarity of being stuck at the Impasse has a perverse sense of comfort simply because it has become your "normal". You are so used to avoiding feeling anxious or feeling sad. Comfortably uncomfortable is one way to think of this. When you recognize that you are still coping with an updated version in the present of a scary historical event from the past, you can then experience rather than avoid the separation anxiety that gets triggered in the replay. If you can do this, you are at the entryway of stopping your chronic hunger for something that only exists in your mind.

Recognizing your Impasse is your wake-up call to become aware of and experience your separation from your loving self or higher mind. When you begin the journey of reconnecting to your spiritual perspective, you will know that you are not abandoned and therefore never really alone.

Take Action: Breakthrough!

1. It is now time to think about and write down some situation where you found yourself feeling particularly uncomfortable or that evoked a body reaction, anger, or fear in you. Use the space below for this exercise.

_____

_____

_____

_____

_____

_____

2. Recognize when you are performing in an updated version of an historical scene (something that happened to you in the past) and allow yourself to experience rather than avoid the unpleasant separation anxiety that gets triggered in the replay. You need to experience your legitimate anxiety in order to heal.

_____

_____

_____

_____

_____

_____

3. Now write in your journal the personal historical story that comes to mind for you.

_____

_____

_____

_____

_____

4. After you have finished journaling, say to yourself, "Something is getting triggered in me. And it is activating in my own historical neurocircuitry. It's okay that this is going on for me. I will not judge it. I will remain calm so that I may identify what is coming to the surface. By identifying and getting conscious of it, I will take better care of myself. Also, I don't have to react the way I did as a child. I am an adult now and have other choices. I do not have to distract myself from this upset in order to prevail. Instead, I need to feel it, move through it, and remember that my incident was in the past and does not have to hold any meaning for me in the present. It is powerless over me today."

5. Write down the subjects that trigger your impasses: (Some examples might be childhood violence, molestation, abandonment, corporal punishment, divorce, death of a family member, death of a child, moving, an angry father/mother, a passive mother/father, peer rejection, failure at something we attempted, bullying, cheating, accidents, foul weather, illness, addictions, neglect, certain words, the parental "look", etc.)

_____

_____

_____

_____

_____

_____

6. Put your Impasse into words in your journal. Remember, your Impasse contains your <u>memory</u> of the event, your <u>feelings</u> about the event when it happened and how you <u>judged</u> yourself or others involved in light of the event.

_____

_____

_____

_____

_____

_____

No one knows your Impasse better than you. Develop an inner awareness of your Impasse and make friends with it. Don't avoid it any more. Right now we ask you to recognize it so you can move forward and think peacefully about it.

CHAPTER THREE

Cutting the Ball and Chain that Weighs You Down

Step Three: Release Your Past

When we remain attached to a painful part of the past, we cannot connect to our innocent spiritual self or higher thinking. This type of higher thinking helps us stay peacefully centered in the here and now. Having recognized your personal Impasse around food, and having made the decision to no longer retreat from it through binging and overeating, you can now begin to access your higher mind or spiritual self.

In the beginning this might be experienced as a challenge because you are in the throes of separation anxiety at the time you call upon yourself to ...."Just Stop Eating That!" However, what is different now is that you can take a leap of faith that in stopping this distraction, you can find your way back to your spirit, the part of you that feels broken from an earlier point in your life. As we give fear over to our higher thinking, we receive spiritual traits in ourselves such as courage, trust, hope, forgiveness and faith.

The Power of a Memory

Take a moment to define the past. It's commonly thought of as *the time before or time gone by*. What does that mean? The past is a span of time. Is that tangible? We don't think so. Your memories of time gone by are all that really exist now and they exist only in your mind. Memories are not really the past; they are only perceptions of it. Have you ever experienced an event with another person where you were present for the same period of time in that shared situation, and later, you both recalled the incident differently? It is important to realize that *what* you remember is far less impacting than *how* you remember. The historical action is over. It is only your judgment of it that actually remains.

This may be a prudent time to think about how you remember the use of food in your early life. What memories does the concept of food conjure up for you? Did your family dine together every evening? If so, how were the family dynamics during the meal? Was it a time of exchanging pleasurable conversation, or was

there a lot of tension and fighting, either aloud or silent-
ly? Think about the concept of "breaking bread". Was it
a positive force in that it reinforced a sense of community? Or was it a time when loved ones come together to air
their dirty laundry, fuss and fight? Did you come from
a large family where when by the time the serving plate
came to you, there was something left? Or was there
no food at all? Or were you one of the group of children
who would sit alone at a table for hours after the meal was
over with a plate of beets and liver staring you in the face?

*It is important to realize that what you
remember is far less impacting than
how you remember.*

Did you eat your dinner alone? Were you waiting for
someone to fill that empty place but they never showed
up? Did you grab your meals on the run for fuel?
Was food used for nourishment and sustenance? Or, was
it used as a discipline and false sense of comfort? There is
so much to be revealed about your eating challenges
today through understanding the role that food played in
your family of origin.

A parent's memory of family life around food may be
very different from their child's. The parents may remember the family situation to have been positive and healthy
around food, with joyful gatherings. They may see their
roles as very involved, nurturing and caring. The child's

perception may be infinitely different. The child may remember the family events and their relationship with their parents to have been, at times, unsafe. Perhaps when the parents were angry, under the influence, absent either through physical or mental illness, they were perceived by the child as abandoning. This is very frightening to a child, because after all, an abandoned child will die. So what does that child in order to be safe? **Distract him or herself through food. Eating equals safety.** At the time, that may have been true. Today, you are questioning that particular script that repeats in your mind.

Think about this as a possibility. Perhaps the parents were preoccupied with their own lives and the child began to feel abandoned and unloved. Young children do not yet have the cognitive ability or the brain development to rationalize that a parent's unavailability is about the parent and has nothing to do with the child's value. A child of any age thinks the parent's unavailability or abandonment is not because of the parent, but because the child himself is not lovable enough. Now we ask you, who was right in their perception and who was wrong? Neither? Both?

Wake Up From the Nightmare

When this child decides to release the past, he or she understands that the existing memory of any particularly painful historical event was simply one point-of-view. When this same child overcomes or rises above his fear of those upsetting or scary situations, he also relinquishes *his personal judgment* about his lovability in the context of those scary events.

The point is that a perception of your past exists only in your mind and that is all there is left of it. The events themselves are much less meaningful than how you took in the events as they occurred. How you took them in, experienced them, felt about them, processed them, and judged yourself in the context of them is what makes up your perception of them. You have the power to change your perception any time you choose to relinquish judgment of the past. When you relinquish judgment, you have released it.

Remember our friend Don. He was a force-fed child whose Impasse was that he was unlovable and he would be left if he didn't eat. Don worked to release his past by relinquishing his judgment that he was not worthy of his mother's regard, the precursor to his own identity. He was erroneously basing his self-concept on a false belief system. He eventually learned that his mother's need for approval through her food wasn't good, it wasn't bad, it just was, and it had nothing to do with him. Don began to shift his thinking.

When you relinquish judgment,
you have released it.

You certainly recall that Mona's Impasse included seeing herself as invisible and, therefore, inadequate.

She worked to release her past by relinquishing her early judgment that since she went unnoticed, she must not be good enough. She learned that her parents' fascination with her brother wasn't good or bad—it just was.

Shortly after she relinquished her judgment about this aspect of her history, she noticed a heightened awareness of her automatic eating. One day she found herself standing in front of the open refrigerator and this time she asked herself, "Why are you standing here? You are not even hungry!" She closed the door and watered her plants instead. What an interesting exchange! Mona gave her need for nourishing to her plants and felt satisfied.

Mark's Impasse included seeing himself as a big disappointment because he could not cope well after the death of his dad. He relinquished judgment about that time in his life and he realized that his challenge in coping after the death of his dad wasn't either good or bad—it just was. A few days after this realization, Mark started to think and journal about how he wanted to cope with the stress of life and came up with some ideas that were truly resilient. For example, instead of brooding after being reprimanded for tardiness at work, Mark bought himself a new electronic device that pleasantly reminded him of where he needed to be. This allowed Mark to feel quite competent in how he could address his need to be on time.

Some of you have a self-definition that is based on what those who cared for you told you directly or indirectly about who you were. If you were told over and over that you were smart, stupid, industrious, lazy, indecisive, impulsive, headstrong, hard-headed, clumsy, graceful, fat, skinny, a sissy, a jock, etc., these remarks could have become a foundation for your identity and may have gotten in the way of your fulfillment in exploring and discovering *on your own* who you wanted to be and what was important to you. Imagine if you were free of those judgments and intrusions into your development. Who would you be? How might you choose to define yourself? How would you take care of yourself and your body? How would you treat the role of food in your life?

> *Imagine if you were free of those judgments and intrusions into your development.*

Now we realize that there are those of you who are stuck at the Impasse and we hear the balking. "Right, ladies, my mother put the dish of liver in front of me and made me remain at the table for hours until I ate it and you are telling me I have a faulty perception of the event." Yes, your mother did make you sit there for hours with a smelly dish of liver in front of you and it appears she is still doing it, only now, she has your permission to do so. You see, the liver itself no longer exists. The sitting and feeling sad hurt you at the time it happened. It was very painful. Today, only your perception of it remains.

Try to grasp this concept. The liver itself never had any meaning. *The way you felt about yourself at the time it happened imparts the only remaining meaning the liver has.* How did you feel when you were being left alone, at the table, with the liver? Afraid? Sad? Shameful? Angry? What have you done about these feelings? One thing you've done is distract yourself from those feelings by eating all the stuff that tastes much better than liver rather than have those feelings so that they may be resolved.

Another possibility is that you haven't been able to release this particular aspect of your past and move forward. You may have swallowed these feelings through binge eating and now remain a slave to keeping them suppressed. This unconscious choice prevents you from truly loving yourself and making higher thinking choices of how you want to take care of yourself. Binge eating, and impulsive and distracting behavior, prevents you from acknowledging and respecting the legitimate feeling part of your life experience. Instead of having your negative feelings, these feelings are having you.

Once again we repeat: relinquish your judgment of a scary memory and you have released that memory. Being forced to eat food to prove your lovability by your mother was bad when she did it, but it isn't bad now, because it isn't happening now. It just was.

You may tend to blame your parents for the misery you continue to experience as an adult. You are at risk to see yourself as a victim and start to believe that unless your parents fix it or apologize, you remain forever at the mercy of their crimes. That is when you turn your attention to food to distract yourself from your feelings of fear and powerlessness. But are you powerless now?

Consider this. It's not about your parents anymore. Now it is all about you and your perceptions of them, and yourself in relation to them. Continuing to blame or judge parents, or anyone else for that matter, is just another distraction from your chronic fear and sadness.

Mona could spend a lifetime blaming her mother and father for abandoning her and causing her great fear and anxiety. She could blame them for her obesity and for taking away her childhood innocence and giftedness. Or, she could choose to forgive them and in so doing, release *herself* from the stronghold these memories have on her life.

From Victim To Victorious

How do you change your fearful perceptions of past events so that you can release them and reconnect to the power of your spirit? Through forgiveness, that's how.

Forgiveness, **the relinquishment of judgment followed by a thought of peace,** is the path to recovery from binge eating and the consequential cycle of suffering. Without forgiveness, you will always be stopped at your Impasse, finding it impossible to connect to your spirit and your higher mind. For Mark, it was realizing that he was always deserving of loving parents, even though he lost his father to death and his mother to grief and having to work. He recognized that as long as he carried his childhood fear in the here and now, he could never move forward to realize his healthy and higher self.

*...the relinquishment of judgment followed
by a thought of peace...*

As long as Mark kept swallowing his fear in food, he hated himself and continued to feed the problem. Mark worked on forgiving himself for thinking he was a disappointment. He forgave his father for dying so young. He forgave his mother for having to provide money instead of parenting.

How do you relinquish judgment of someone else or yourself for a painful mistake? Ask yourself this question, "How would I know this differently if I considered it from a position of love rather than fear?" In other words, "How would my spirit have me know this?" The pain of a scary childhood event can be overwhelming from a position of fear. It can also disappear when you release it with forgiveness.

Sorrowful Suzanne

Suzanne was crisis nurse in the neo-natal unit of a major city hospital. Suzanne would work any shift, all shifts, as long as she could remain at the station that was adjacent to the kitchen. When you looked at Suzanne's work area, it was usually covered with snack wrappers of all kinds. Her pockets were stuffed with patient snacks like pudding, applesauce and bags of chips. Her binge eating had progressed to the point where she thought nothing of eating while interacting with parents who were anxiety-ridden about the well-being of their infants.

Suzanne was an excellent nurse and a compassionate person, but her compulsive overeating had crossed over into every area of her life. When she went in for her yearly review, her supervisor gently told her that her preoccupation with food was intrusive into her job. She strongly recommended that Suzanne get some help.

Suzanne came to see us feeling quite worried about the future of her job. One of our first observations was that she appeared to have no boundaries around food. We were much less concerned about the food and much more concerned about the boundaries. And so we asked her about how her boundaries were treated as a child. The tears flowed.

Sadly, she had been sexually molested by her brother three years her senior, beginning at the age of 9. Initially, she told her mother who was rarely at home because she worked in the family business. Her mother apathetically responded to her appeal for help by stating, "Your brother is a developing young man. You just better keep away from him. I've seen how you walk around the house in those short shorts. What do you expect? How do you expect him to respond with your parading around like that?" Suzanne felt blamed and ashamed. Her Impasse, from that historical event, was that she must be unlovable and unworthy of her mother's protection. She felt afraid and sad that without it, she could die.

In light of that abandonment, Suzanne had to find a way to ward off her brother's scary advances.

She turned to food and found that if she was fat, he wouldn't pay attention to her. Additionally, if she was in the kitchen, he would tend to leave her alone. Suzanne went from 60 pounds to 112 pounds in one year. Her weight exponentially increased until at 25, she topped the scales and 230 pounds.

Once Suzanne recognized her impasse of fear and sadness, we began the powerful work of forgiveness. Suzanne had to forgive her parents for their apathy and failure to protect her; she had to forgive her brother for his repetitive sexual assaults; and she had to forgive herself for believing that she in some way was responsible for this horrible situation.

Her parents' abandonment of her wasn't good or bad—it just was. She deserved their protection and intervention. She didn't get it. Not because she didn't deserve it, but because they were caught up with the minutiae of their own busy lives. Forgiving her brother was a bit more of a challenge, because his acts of sexual assault were so heinous. To achieve this act of forgiveness, Suzanne created a letter to her brother where she expressed her righteous indignation at his behavior.

Suzanne then began the ongoing work of forgiving herself by realizing that she had developed a faulty perception of her value and lovability. She corrected this perception and took a good look at how she was failing to protect herself by carrying an extra 100 pound of weight. At the time of this writing, Suzanne was down to 158 pounds and was the discharge nurse in a weight loss clinic.

Forgiveness is for people, not for actions. When you are faced with an awful mistake, be it your own or someone else's, it would be far more effective to forgive yourself and/or the other and give the mistake over to your higher mind. This relinquishment invites wisdom in to handle the problem. Imagine freeing yourself from the ball and chain of binge eating. You can **Just Stop Eating That** with the goal of forgiveness.

Your unconscious attachment to some parts of your past prohibit you from neurologically bridging to the higher mind or spiritual self, which is the most powerful and peaceful part of you. When that part of you is present, you can stay peacefully centered in the here and now. Having identified your Impasse and deciding no longer to retreat from it, you can now begin to mend the break in your spiritual bridge and forge new neural pathways to higher thinking which allows you to make healthier choices.

By releasing your painful perception of the past, you can stop protecting an historical fear and heal your connection to hope and peacefulness. You are now beginning to successfully connect or bridge to your higher thinking and access the power of your spiritual self. This will empower you to eat to live rather than live to eat.

In releasing the past you must remember that your memories don't equal the past. *What* you remember is far less impacting than *how* you remember it. The historical action itself is over. It is only your judgment of yourself and others in its context that remains. For example, if you have a memory of being disciplined by an aggressive parent, there may be a childlike part of you that remembers this event with embarrassment or shame. You may believe, in some way that you were not worthy of receiving love. The memory itself is far less damaging than your perception or judgment of who you are in light of it.

So, think of this possibility. When you are just with you. Bang!! A trigger is tripped. Loneliness puts you at your Impasse, makes you anxious and keeps you stuck in fear. You binge eat to relieve the discomfort, even if only for a few minutes. Then, you cycle right back to feeling isolated and lonely all over again.

In releasing the past you must remember that your memories don't equal the past.

Take some time now and reflect upon some memory that has resulted in a negative self-judgment. It does not necessarily need to be as dramatic as some of the examples used in this book in order to illustrate a particular point. Maybe someone in your past contributed to the story of your identity by helping you to believe you are something that you would prefer not to be. You can shift your perception of that memory right now by stating, "That memory is not bad. It just is."

Now ask yourself, "How do I feel about myself in relation to food?" If the answer is fat, unlovable, unattractive, unhappy, exhausted and sad, then abusing food is not sustaining you. Releasing the past through the relinquishment of judgment begins breaking down your Impasse and opening the pathways to your spirit or your higher thinking. Now, you are ready to use thoughts of peace to **Just Stop Eating That!** when you are being challenged by fear.

Take Action: Freedom Through Forgiveness

1. Review and list the historical events that you identified as Impasses.

_____

_____

_____

_____

_____

_____

2. Correlate the feelings you had with those particular Impasse memories and write them down. (Painful memories might typically elicit a feeling of sadness, embarrassment, shame, disappointment, anger and/or fear. These feelings, unaddressed, may generate a personal sense of inadequacy in you which can be mirrored in the type of person you attract.)

_____

_____

_____

_____

_____

_____

3. List the judgments or negative thoughts you made about yourself or others around these Impasse events. For example: "I was a bad girl because my father was always angry", or "I was unlovable because no one paid attention to me."

_____

_____

_____

_____

_____

_____

4. In order to rid yourself of these judgments and faulty beliefs, you now need to exchange your fear for forgiveness.

a. Admit you have the fear. Write down what you are afraid of (e.g. I have a fear of not being good enough, of being stupid, embarrassed, etc.).

_____

_____

_____

_____

_____

_____

b. Take personal responsibility for the role your memory is playing in your life and decide what it is you want to create around this memory (e.g., healing, peace, calmness, closure, release or forgiveness versus resentment, anger, hostility, grievance, continued pain, vengeance, depression, anxiety or physical illness).

_____

_____

_____

_____

_____

_____

c. Realize the negative judgment or faulty thinking you associate with the historical event and on the person or persons in the event with you. List these counterproductive thoughts, perceptions and judgments.

_____

_____

_____

_____

_____

_____

d. Remove all descriptors (adjectives or adverbs) that depict the event. For example rather than say, "My father was a disgusting drunk and I hated him!, say instead, "My father drank too much and sometimes I felt afraid of him."

_____

_____

_____

_____

_____

_____

e. Remove all your judgments, unconsciously made at an earlier time, from the description of the event. Commit to exchange your fear around this event with forgiveness; forgiveness of yourself and forgiveness of the others who were involved. **You do not have to forgive the event itself. The event may not have been okay.** You are forgiving yourself and the other people involved so **you can be released**. Remember, this forgiveness is not for them- it is for **you** to be free. It is through your forgiveness of the other person that you can be released from a painful past.

_____

_____

_____

_____

_____

_____

f. Write in the space below, I forgive... (e.g. my father for being an alcoholic) and I forgive myself for... (e.g. believing I wasn't lovable enough for him to stop drinking).

_____

_____

_____

_____

_____

_____

5. Forgiveness is for people not for actions. For example, spanking is an action. Because you were spanked doesn't mean you were bad. Maybe you engaged in behavior that was unacceptable. That doesn't mean you are unacceptable. You made a mistake, you're not a mistake. What stands in your way when you think about forgiveness (e.g., some people see themselves as justified in carrying grievances.)?

_____

_____

_____

_____

_____

_____

In deciding to release the past, you can move from fear to forgiveness. Forgiveness is the release of judgment followed by peaceful thoughts. You can now remember that in light of a painful memory, you remain worthy of compassion and regard. Remember, it is not only someone else's compassion and regard that counts. Your compassion and regard for yourself is paramount to your recovery. The thoughts of peace will now serve you in your next step, responding to fear.

CHAPTER FOUR

Satisfy Your Hunger for Serenity

Step Four: Responding to Your Fear

The Limbic: How Low Can You Go?

Responding and reacting are two different behaviors. **Overeating is a reacting behavior. Eating a nourishing meal or snack is a responding behavior.** These behaviors originate from different places in your brain. Reacting involves little or no thought. It is automatic and falls into the neurocircuitry of your lower brain or limbic functioning.

Reactions are defensive in nature and based on your primitive instincts of fight, flight or freeze. You react when you have a need to protect yourself. Sometimes this is desirable. If your body is starving and needs fuels, your basic instinct will be to eat. This is a good thing. When your body is starving, binge eating would not remedy the situation. Instead, you would hydrate with water and slowly begin to ingest small amounts of nourishment, allowing your body to metabolize the food for energy, rather than binging and stress your body by making it store the excessive calories as fat.

We want to remind you again of the brain science involved in order for you to **Just Stop Eating That!** Your limbic system is meant to intervene in emergency situations where you are immediately threatened. Remember that the limbic system was evolutionarily important for survival of the fittest. People were instinctually driven to hunt, gather and eat so that they would survive and reproduce. Even though some countries are struggling to feed their people, most of us are no longer living in a society where we need to be driven to eat! The irony is that you have to eat in order to survive, so you are faced with the challenges of food every day!

We need for you to accept that you have gone limbic with your eating. How low can you go?! Reactive eating will destroy your emotional and physical well-being. It is devastating to your spiritual health to reactively eat and then suffer the shame and self-loathing that accompanies this vicious cycle. It is now time to bridge up to your higher thinking when making decisions about eating.

The thoughtful preparation of an action is called responding. How do you respond in times of anxiety? Do you try to swallow your feelings with food? Do try to fill a void with food? Do you ever satisfy your hunger? Do you even know what truly sustains you? If you learn to respond, rather than react when you think about eating, you will be able to remain present and accountable for what you chose to put in your mouth.

The thoughtful preparation of an action is called responding.

Responding to fear rather than reacting to it supports your release of the past. Once you have relinquished negative self-judgment originating from early relationships with food, you are empowered to stay internally peaceful and better able make satisfying menu choices.

You have already committed to let go of the past. You have committed to no longer perceive yourself as a victim of it. When fear is triggered you can now recognize that you are at your Impasse. You can choose to rise above your separation anxiety and remember that you are not abandoned and that you are not alone. With that in mind, you are not looking for food to complete you. You now look for healthy food choices and creativity in deciding what truly nourishes your spirit and holistic sense of well-being. You will discover how to be present for yourself in a way that addresses your moods, your needs, your thoughts, your desires, your intentions and your goals. This is called bringing out the best in yourself.

When you begin to respond to these old unconscious fears, you empower yourself to show up. Your precious, spiritual self is showing. Not your fear-driven, scared little child. Your spiritual self is confidently showing up with authenticity, courage, peace and faith in your ability to truly take care of yourself.

Have you ever felt afraid or insecure and used food to make yourself feel better? What is that fear about? Why are you afraid? Take some time right now and think about the answers to these questions and write them down.

The relationship with food is a mirror of the relationship you create with yourself.

How much and how often do you eat so you don't have to feel the fear? Emotional reactive eating occurs as a result of poor impulse control which is in the limbic system. Your immediate impulse is to get away from the scary feeling because it is unpleasant. If you remember, our Impasses consist of the unpleasant feeling of fear and sadness. You impulsively turn to binge eating which gives fear power over your logical ability to make healthier decisions around food and eating. You unconsciously abandon yourself when you spend all your time focusing and reacting to food. If you are not eating, you are thinking about when you are going to eat, what you are going to eat, with whom you are going to eat, and the list goes on and on. This dishonors what you are really feeling.

The relationship with food is a mirror of the relationship you create with yourself. You are relating to food in a hateful way because you are abusing it, and in turn, abusing yourself. Your limbic system may tell you to eat, but it's your higher mind that can help you decide what, how much and when you are going to eat.

React with Food—Respond with Peace

Below are examples of Reactive & Responsive Eating.

REACTIVE EATING	RESPONSIVE EATING
Eating an entire pizza by yourself	Eating a slice or two of pizza
Driving through numerous fast food restaurants and eating everything in the car	Selecting a healthy fast food choice, taking it home and eating it at your table
Eating all day long as a part of multi-tasking	Taking several breaks and eating several small meals during these breaks
Wolfing down your food without experiencing it	Eating slowly to experience taste, texture and healthy digestion
Eating even though you are full	Figuring out what you are truly hungry for
Eating when you feel stressed	Practicing stress release before eating
Coming home from work or school and immediately eating anything you can find	Taking time to unwind, transition, get comfortable and then prepare your meal
Eating when you are angry	Having your anger responsibly
Not eating all day and binging all night	Having six small meals during the day
Having multiple servings of food at holiday meals	Having one serving and always leave some food in your dish
Eating an container of ice cream or entire bag of chips/cookies/candy	Having a small serving
Stocking your pantry with Junk Food	Shopping with a list and not feeling hungry as an exercise to reinforce healthy eating
Eating when you are depressed	Feeling and respecting your depression
Eating a light meal with others and then going home to binge	Coming out of the closet and gaining the support of others

Frequenting all-you-can-eat buffets	Staying away from unhealthy environments
Eating your meal plus what others leave in their plates	Respecting boundaries and eating only your own food
Eating something so not to waste it	Nice try! Stop your denial
Eating out all the time	Being mindful and preparing a meal

Stop, Look, and Listen

If you acknowledge your fear, instead of running from it, then you can respond rather than react to it. Responding is a discipline and it requires a lot of practice to become good at it. **Responding to fear is best developed by following three behavioral steps: Stop, Look and Listen**.

Do you remember this phrase being taught to you as a child when learning to cross the street? Some streets may be easier to cross than others. How many streets have you crossed where you never bothered to stop, look and listen? At some of the scary intersections, you could be easily mowed down if you didn't adhere to the rule. When you find yourself at a frightening emotional intersection, the rule of responding is to Stop! Look! And Listen!

Let's start with **Stop**. Identify what will become your personal red light. When you are dating or in a relationship with someone and you become triggered, your historical fear becomes activated and you may not recognize this as fear. Your red light might be a gnawing feeling in the pit of your stomach; the hair might stand up on the back of your neck; you might turn to a bad habit; you might even feel yourself becoming depressed. You may become very perfectionistic or you might procrastinate and avoid taking care of important things in your own life. Your work life might start to suffer or you may start ignoring your children. You have gotten yourself so deep into managing or fixing the other, you don't even notice it anymore. It's like breathing out and breathing in.

Identify what will become your
personal red light.

Ironically, you will find yourself at a place where your distraction becomes your greatest reminder to respond, rather than react, to what is going on. Pay attention to yourself for a change!

Don was able to identify his red light as the times when he felt himself looking for the approval of others rather than looking inward to himself. Now that Don had recognized his Impasse, he became aware of a gnawing feeling in his gut when he was seeking outside approval. He stopped and noticed the feeling. He looked inside and saw an innocent little boy. He heard that little boy ask for self-acceptance and self-regard. Instead of binge-eating as an ineffective way to quell the gnawing feeling, he did something that he could feel really good about—he researched a bit on the Internet and then he picked up the phone and made a few calls.

Don decided to give what he was looking to get. He worked to become a Big Brother and a positive role model for a needy child. Don became so involved in the program that food really took a back seat in his life. Without even trying, he lost 18 pounds. His relationship with food shifted into something healthy and positive. He still had the gnawing feeling every now and again, but he responded, rather than react to it. Rather than reactively binge-eat, he would choose to do something he could feel truly good about instead.

Mona found her red light to be spending too much time alone. Her heightened consciousness helped her to stop for a second when she was in the house all day long and look inside. She saw a sweet little girl who said, "Please see me!" Mona listened to the request of her child-like self and instead of overeating as a way to isolate and remain 'invisible', she decided to take herself to an Overeaters Anonymous meeting. She stood up at the podium and let herself be seen. Everyone at the meeting gave her recognition. Now that Mona had recognized her Impasse of invisibility, she could respond to her tendency to be reclusive instead of reactively eat, hibernating in the house and invisible to the world.

How ironic that Mona's Impasse of being invisible was something she breathed life into every day through overeating. The bigger Mona got, the less frequently she went out and so she had very little social connection. Once Mona starting utilizing the **Stop, Look and Listen** technique, she began to change the nature of her relationship with food. She got connected with others who wanted to **Just Stop Eating That!** Her visibility in the world of weight loss helped her to drop over eighty pounds in four months!

Mark found his red light to be when he heard himself saying "yes" to things he really didn't want to do. He hated to be a disappointment to others, but his recognition of his Impasse helped him realize that he couldn't be all things to all people all the time, without abandoning himself. Mark's red light became his agreement to put someone else's needs before his own. When he started to do that, he would stop and look inside. He heard a charming child plead, "Please don't leave me if I disappoint you!" The first dozen or so times Mark heard this inner truth, he would get choked up and his eyes would well up with tears. He would remind that little inside guy that he was no disappointment; that he never was and never would be!

As soon Mark starting saying, "No", things really shifted for him. He started to feel more confident and his self-esteem improved. Well, what do you know!? He hired a personal trainer who really helped him to learn how to take care of himself and discern the times when it was good for him to say "yes" or "no". Mark is enjoying life and has lost a carload of weight.

Suzanne found her red light to be a wrapper or a "treat" in her desk drawer or pocket. Or, when food shopping, she purchased food that she knew she wouldn't eat, just to have it! Now that Suzanne understood that this trail of "crumbs" could lead her back to her preciousness, she would stop, look inside to the innocent little girl she was and listen. "Please don't let them hurt me!" Tears streamed down her cheeks during these fleeting moments of **Stop, Look and Listen**. She heard the plea for protection and she committed to herself that she would fully show up to protect herself in any scary situation.

Suzanne noticed how her thinking shifted around food. Protecting herself translated into making healthy, nourishing eating choices. She began to understand how she could endanger herself through repetitive binging. Suzanne began to develop a strategy for eating that kept her safe: physically, emotionally, and spiritually. She became very involved with health and nutrition and eventually became head-nurse in a weight loss clinic. She also became involved in Neighborhood Crime Watch and worked with her neighbors and friends to increase safety in their community.

You are gaining courage and so you are ready to respond to the fears that children avoid feeling in order to survive.

You may have noticed by now that every Impasse is driven by the feelings of fear and sadness. When you release your past you are free to feel these legitmate feelings that hooked you into distracting yourself by eating too much. You are gaining courage and so you are ready to respond to the fears that children avoid feeling in order to survive. As an adult, you are not defenseless. You can stand present for yourself in the here and now because you are thinking more clearly.

Take Action: Facing Your Fear

1. Stop, Look and Listen

Do you remember this phrase being taught to you as a child when you were learning to cross the street? Some streets are easier to cross than others. At some of the dangerous intersections, you could easily be mowed down if you didn't adhere to the rule. When you find yourself at a scary emotional intersection in your work, the rule of responding is to **Stop, Look and Listen**.

Stop. Identify what will become your personal red light. What was once a burden in your distraction from fear can now serve you as a blessing as it signals that something is being triggered for you. Simply stop. What is your adult distraction when you feel afraid? BINGE EATING! Keep in mind you could have more than one distraction.

Look. Look inside, become introspective and think about what is being triggered in your history. Acknowledge it. Honor it. Relinquish judgment about yourself and others involved. Think peacefully about it. Forgive it. For example, if you think you are protecting yourself from someone crossing your boundaries by eating and creating a thick wall of fat, think again. Do you never want to be physically close with someone? Wouldn't you rather find a new way to negotiate your boundaries so they are intact with a balance of give and take? If you stop the binge eating that has masked your pain, you have now freed yourself to look inward and see the real truth as to what is happening.

Listen. Listen to your inner voice and your inner truth. What would you really want for yourself if you weren't so scared and afraid? Write it down.

2. Write about a time when you had an upsetting experience and then overate voraciously. As you write it, you can listen peacefully to your inner story and remember that this story is about *you* and not about the event, or anyone else in the story. The upset belongs to you and you need to be accountable for it. Then, realize you deserve to forgive, to be forgiven and to be more patient with yourself and the others involved. Write your story using "I" statements and conclude with the statement: "May this story rest in peace".

_____

_____

_____

_____

_____

_____

_____

_____

_____

_____

_____

_____

_____

_____

_____

_____

_____

_____

_____

3. Practice the two forgiveness steps of relinquishing judgment followed by peaceful thoughts. In the space below, make a forgiveness list for hurts you have incurred in your life. Every story is an opportunity for practicing forgiveness which has been coined for centuries as being divine.

_____

_____

_____

_____

_____

_____

_____

_____

4. Make a list of all the people you want to forgive and also include the things for which you wish to be forgiven.

_____

_____

_____

_____

_____

_____

_____

_____

_____

This practice is universally healing and the person doing the forgiving is successfully bridging or connecting to his/her higher mind, creating new-found hope, faith and trust in the ability to form a healthy relationship with food.

CHAPTER FIVE

Living With a Full Heart

Step Five: Reconnecting to Your Higher Mind

This is the most rewarding part of the process. There is nothing you have to do. There is nothing you have to figure out. Simply let your mind be still. Now that you are no longer distracted, anxious, worried or fearful, you have opened the way to clear your mind and connect to your higher self where you receive the characteristics or traits of higher mind thinking. This allows you to bring these traits into your relationship with food and attract those with similar traits.

Creative Spiritual Practice

Now that you are no longer distracted and can let your mind be still, you are empowered to start engaging in some practice which will allow wisdom, calming and peaceful thoughts into your relationship with food. Let your mind receive and connect to them. Engage in activities to strengthen the connection, such as:

- meditation
- prayer
- nature hikes
- gardening
- 12-step programs
- playing sports
- running
- engaging in the arts
- reading
- journaling
- playing games
- expressing gratitude
- yoga
- joining an encouragement group
- dancing
- cooking healthy food

You'll meet other great people through these activities who are also invested in connecting this way. Develop a spirituality or peace plan, something that you will do daily, weekly, monthly to clear your mind and allow the spiritual traits to come into your thinking. We recommend utilizing a wellness planner to help keep you on track. Look on the last page of this book for our wellness planner recommendation.

Let us revisit our friends who went through the five simple steps. Franny the Freshman graduated college with honors. After her dramatic weight loss, she worked with others to help them face their fears and drop the pounds. She decided to get a graduate degree in nutrition, educating and helping people to be mindful of what they put in their body. Franny follows an exercise program like a religion, in that she practices it faithfully. Typically, after a good workout she will spend the rest of the morning with her exercise group, socializing and sharing a healthy breakfast.

...utilizing a wellness planner to
help keep you on track.

Hungry Hannah, whose warring parents focused on their mutual embarrassment around her weight, moved away and joined Overeaters Anonymous. This 12-step recovery program resonated for Hannah and she developed a strong network of support. Her relationship with her sponsor was very healing for her and she had friends who shared the same values and she did.

Mac N' Cheese Mona became involved with Meals on Wheels where she helped the poor and sick to receive a friendly visit and a home-cooked meal. Funny, Mona reported that while she was working to deliver food, she never felt hungry. She spent her free time at the lake where she had a small cabin and enjoyed the scents and sounds of nature.

Mouthful Mark realized that in order to maintain his spiritual perspective, he needed to become a part of a community where he truly believed he belonged. He joined the horticultural society and learned everything there was to know about plants and flowers. He eventually opened an extremely successful landscape architecture firm and thoroughly enjoyed his hearty appetite for beautiful plants.

Dining Don became a Buddhist. This worked for him particularly because fasting was something that appealed to him. Letting go of food helped him to form a new relationship with it; one that was completely different from his historical experience. He met a lovely Buddhist woman and they married and had four children.

Sorrowful Suzanne went into therapy and experienced Eye Movement Desensitization Restructuring (EMDR) for her traumatic memories of sexual abuse. Once she experienced trauma relief, she was able to become aware of her eating triggers so that she could **Stop! Look! (within) and Listen** to her story with compassion and a peaceful heart. Initially, she lost a chunk of weight and still struggles with the last 25 pounds, but she is determined to take care of herself and stay the path.

Please take plenty of time to think about activities that would truly be a fit for your spiritual growth. Any experience that is uplifting for you will work. Also remember that any spiritual practice requires repetition. That is why it is called a practice.

Take Action: How Will You Feed Your Soul?

List some loving qualities you want to nurture within yourself, so that you can see them mirrored in the person you attract.

_____

_____

_____

_____

_____

_____

_____

_____

_____

Write down all the things that you wish you had the time to do and haven't been able to fit into your schedule.

_____

_____

_____

_____

_____

_____

_____

_____

_____

Make 5 affirmations that you can repeat—one for each day of the work week. For example:

- I am going to be more tolerant and patient.

- I want to be intimate with my own feelings so that I can be accountable for them in my relationships

- I am grateful for the blessings I have and the love I can give.

- I will be introspective today. I will think of any upsetting situations that have occurred so far and address them with the techniques I have learned.

- Today I will nurture myself and my partner.

- This week there have been satisfying and taxing experiences in my relationships. I have learned some important things about myself and my partner. I will use this information to help us to grow.

- I have stayed in the present and not allowed my past to dictate what I attract into my life today.

- I have not been distracted with inappropriate behaviors. I have replaced fear with faith.

Now, write your own:

1. _____

_____

_____

2. _____

_____

_____

3. _____

_____

_____

4. _____

_____

_____

5. _____

_____

_____

Commit to follow through with your plan. Mark the date you'll start on your calendar and schedule it in pen. Use a wellness planner to stay motivated and on track.

We recommend "The 9 Daily Habits of Healthy People" by Melanie Lane, MD.

This is just the start of a very meaningful journey. We wish you well and we know that you will **Just Stop Eating That!**

Ellie and Vicki

The Five Steps of the Rapid Advance Process

RELINQUISHMENT of JUDGMENT	THOUGHT OF PEACE
1. **Reveal Your History**	*It happened.* It was
2. **Recognize Your Impasse**	*It is still happening.* It is.
3. **Release Your Past**	*I can forgive.* I can.
4. **Respond to Your Fear**	*I stop and look within.* I know.
5. **Reconnect to Your Spirit**	*I find myself.* I am.

ABOUT THE AUTHORS

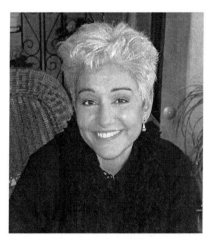

Ellie Izzo, PhD, LPC

Ellie has been in clinical practice for over 30 years. She also serves as a trainer, Divorce Coach and Child Specialist in Collaborative Divorce cases. She developed the Rapid Advance Process, a standardized five-session brief model of counseling that was presented at the American Counseling Association convention in Atlanta in 1997 and with Vicki Carpel Miller in Honolulu in 2008. Ellie is the author of The Bridge To I Am, a self-help book outlining the Rapid Advance Process. Ellie hosted a call-in radio show in Phoenix and served as Self-Help

Editor for a nationally syndicated trade magazine. She runs several ongoing groups called the Encouragers where people meet to offer each other peace, support and acceptance.

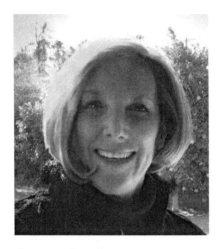

Vicki Carpel Miller, BSN, MS, LMFT

Vicki Carpel Miller is a licensed Marriage and Family Therapist in clinical practice for over 20 years. Vicki was instrumental in bringing Collaborative Divorce to Arizona and functions as a Divorce Coach and Child Specialist in Collaborative Divorce cases. She specializes in the treatment of Vicarious Trauma, the Rapid Advance Process, the practice of Collaborative Divorce and other divorce-related issues such as blended family and stepfamily issues. Vicki is internationally recognized as a trainer with the Collaborative Divorce Training Team.

Vicki and Ellie are co-founders of the Collaborative Divorce Institute and the Vicarious Trauma Institute. Their offices are located in Scottsdale, Arizona.

More books from HCI Press at unHookedBooks.com

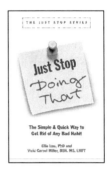

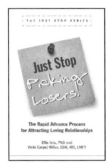

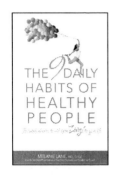

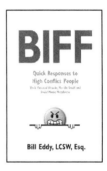

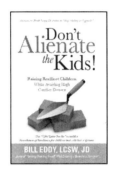

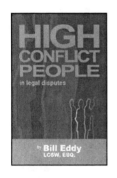

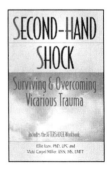

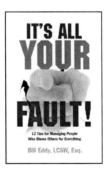

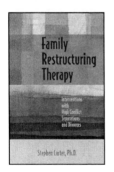

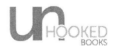

Available from unHookedBooks.com

To order, call 480-420-6355 or visit our online bookstore at unHookedBooks.com.

Visa, MasterCard, Amex
(prices subject to change without notice)

CPSIA information can be obtained at www.ICGtesting.com
Printed in the USA
BVOW011941121011

273506BV00001B/8/P